The Female Sexual Response Cycle

A Guide to Understanding Your Body and Boosting Your Sex Drive

Dr Philip Barker

Table of Contents

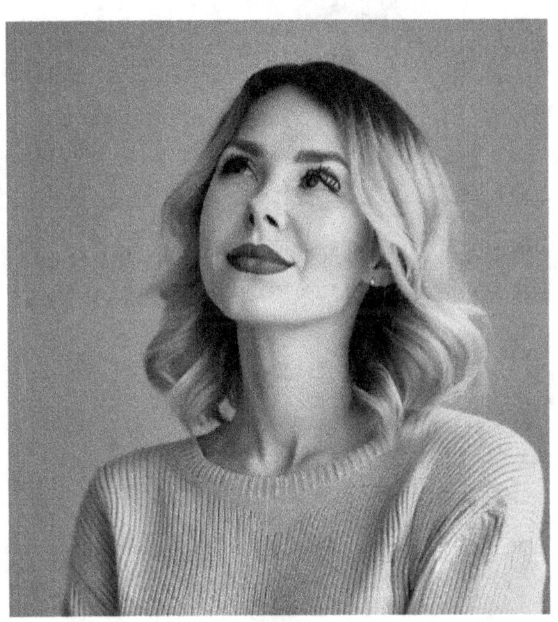

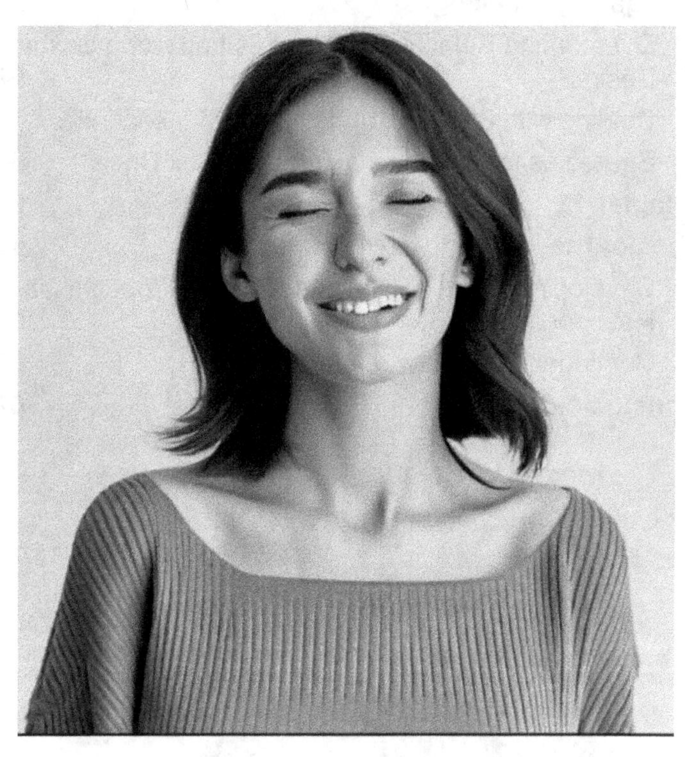

Introduction

Have you ever wondered about the intricate workings of your own body and its remarkable capacity for pleasure? Imagine possessing the knowledge to unlock the secrets of your desires, to ignite your passion, and to cultivate a profound connection with your own sexuality. Welcome to a journey of self-discovery unlike any other, a journey that will empower you to understand and embrace your body's responses, while boosting your sexual drive and transforming your intimate experiences.

In a world where discussions about sexuality are often shrouded in mystery and misinformation, this book stands as a beacon of clarity and empowerment. This book invites you to delve into the depths of your own sensual landscape, unraveling the complexities of desire, arousal, orgasm, and beyond. Whether you're seeking to enhance your sexual well-being, nurture your self-confidence, or foster deeper connections with your partner(s), this guide offers the knowledge and tools to help you achieve your goals.

Gone are the days of uncertainty and shame. This book takes you on a transformative journey, illuminating the physiological, psychological, and emotional dimensions of your sexual response. From the initial spark of desire to the crescendo of pleasure, and even into the afterglow of satisfaction, you'll gain insights that will forever change the way you approach your body and its incredible potential.

Prepare to embark on an odyssey of discovery and empowerment, a journey that embraces diversity, challenges taboos, and fosters inclusivity.

If you're ready to awaken your curiosity, unleash your desires, and transform your relationship with your own body, then this book is your gateway. Let the pages ahead be your companions on a journey of empowerment and discovery, a journey that promises to leave you informed, inspired, and eager to embrace your sexuality with newfound confidence. Your body's responses are a treasure waiting to be unlocked, and this book is your key. Get ready to embark on a path of self-discovery that will forever change the way you perceive yourself and your capacity for pleasure.

Chapter 1

Foundation of Female Sexual Response

Phases of the Female Sexual Response Cycle

Welcome to the heart of understanding your body's most intimate mechanisms, the Female Sexual Response Cycle. Within you lies a symphony of sensations, a complex dance of physiological and psychological shifts that pave the way for pleasure and connection. In this chapter, we'll delve into the four foundational phases that comprise the cycle, illuminating the path from desire to satisfaction.

Phases of the Female Sexual Response Cycle
The Female Sexual Response Cycle is a dynamic and beautifully choreographed sequence of events that unfolds within the female body during sexual activity. Understanding these phases is fundamental to harnessing your sexual potential:

1. *Desire: Unleashing Your Inner Desires*

Desire is the spark that ignites the fires of passion. It's the magnetic force that draws you towards a partner or an idea, the very essence of what makes you yearn for intimate connection. This phase is deeply personal, influenced by a multitude of factors including your physical well-being, emotional state, and the dynamics of your relationships. Cultivating desire involves self-awareness, open communication, and embracing your fantasies. It's about acknowledging what excites you and owning it without shame.

2. *Arousal: Igniting Passion and Physical Readiness*

As desire intensifies, your body begins to respond with a symphony of physiological changes. Blood rushes to your pelvic region, your heart rate increases, and your skin becomes more sensitive to touch. Lubrication and heightened sensitivity pave the way for heightened pleasure. It's during this phase that your body becomes physically primed for sexual activity. The key to embracing arousal lies in relaxation, exploration, and a willingness to embrace sensory experiences without inhibition.

3. Plateau: Reaching the Peak of Pleasure
In the plateau phase, your arousal reaches its zenith. Your body continues to respond to stimulation, intensifying the pleasurable sensations you're experiencing. Muscles contract, heart rate and breathing become more rapid, and you may notice heightened sensitivity in your erogenous zones. It's an exquisite stage of sexual response where time seems to slow, and you become immersed in the sensations of the moment.

4. Orgasm: The Climactic Experience
The orgasm phase is often seen as the crescendo of sexual response. It's a climax of pleasure that can manifest in various ways, from intense waves of sensation to subtle, quivering releases of tension. During orgasm, your brain is flooded with feel-good chemicals like dopamine and oxytocin, providing a powerful sense of euphoria and connection. Learning to embrace and enjoy this phase involves self-acceptance, relaxation, and letting go of any performance pressure.

5. Resolution: Coming Down and Afterglow
As the sexual activity concludes, your body gradually returns to its normal state. The resolution phase involves the gradual dissipation of sexual tension and the return of your body to its baseline.

However, it's important to note that not all sexual encounters end in orgasm, and that's perfectly normal. This phase can still bring a sense of intimacy and emotional connection, often referred to as the "afterglow."

Understanding these phases is just the beginning of your journey. It's an invitation to explore, nurture, and embrace your own sexual response cycle. It's about celebrating your uniqueness and recognizing that your desires are valid, your pleasure matters, and your body is a source of profound joy.

Embrace your desires, learn about your body, and celebrate your unique sexual response cycle. With each passing page of this book, you'll gain insights and tools to enhance your sexual well-being. Get ready to embark on a journey of self-discovery and empowerment that will forever change the way you perceive and engage with your own sexuality.

Chapter 2

The Psychological Aspect

Emotional Factors Influencing Sexual Response

In the intricate interplay of the Female Sexual Response Cycle, the psychological aspect plays a pivotal role. It's a realm where emotions, thoughts, and perceptions converge to shape our sexual experiences. In this chapter, we will delve into the profound influence of psychology on the Female Sexual Response Cycle, exploring emotional factors, body image, self-esteem, and the impacts of stress and anxiety. By understanding these psychological dimensions, you'll gain the keys to unlocking a richer, more fulfilling sexual life.

Sexuality is not just about the body; it's a deeply emotional journey as well. Emotions, both positive and negative, can profoundly influence the Female Sexual Response Cycle.

Desire and Emotions: Desire often takes its cues from our emotional state. Feelings of connection, love, and intimacy can kindle desire, while emotions like anger, resentment, or stress can dampen it. Understanding your emotional landscape and how it intertwines with desire is a crucial step toward a more satisfying sexual life.

Arousal and Emotional Engagement: Arousal is not a mechanical process but a manifestation of emotional engagement. Feeling desired, appreciated, and emotionally connected to your partner(s) can amplify physical arousal. Conversely, unresolved emotional conflicts can hinder it.

Orgasm and Emotional Release: Orgasm is not just a physical climax; it's a release of built-up tension, often accompanied by a surge of positive emotions. Emotional intimacy and trust with your partner(s) can enhance the emotional aspects of orgasm.

Body Image and Self-Esteem

Body image, the way you perceive and feel about your own body, plays a significant role in how you experience your sexuality. It's an aspect that can profoundly affect self-esteem, confidence, and sexual desire.

Self-Perception and Desire: How you perceive your body directly influences your level of desire. A positive body image can boost self-confidence and desire, while negative body image can act as a barrier to intimacy.

Self-Esteem and Intimacy: Self-esteem is the foundation upon which healthy relationships and satisfying sexual experiences are built. Low self-esteem can lead to feelings of inadequacy and inhibit the ability to connect intimately with a partner.

Stress, Anxiety, and Their Effects on Desire and Arousal

The modern world often bombards us with stress and anxiety, which can have profound effects on the Female Sexual Response Cycle.

Stress and Desire: Stress activates the body's "fight or flight" response, diverting resources away from sexual desire. In times of high stress, desire may wane as your body prioritizes survival over reproduction.

Anxiety and Arousal: Anxiety can lead to a state of hyper-vigilance, making it difficult to relax and become aroused. It can also lead to sexual performance anxiety, creating a self-perpetuating cycle of worry.

Coping Strategies: Learning to manage stress and anxiety is essential for a fulfilling sexual life. Techniques like mindfulness, relaxation exercises, and open communication with your partner(s) can be invaluable in reducing the negative impact of these emotions.

Chapter 3

Navigating Hormones and Their Role

Hormonal Changes Across the Sexual Response Cycle

In the symphony of the Female Sexual Response Cycle, hormones are the conductors, orchestrating the intricate dance of desire, arousal, and satisfaction. This chapter takes you on a journey through the hormonal landscape, revealing the profound influence of hormones on sexual experiences. We'll explore the hormonal changes across the Sexual Response Cycle, delve into the impact of the menstrual cycle on desire and arousal, and consider the effects of hormone therapy on sexual drive. By understanding the role of hormones, you'll gain valuable insights into the dynamics of your own body and its responses.

From the quiet whispers of anticipation to the resounding crescendo of orgasm, hormones are the behind-the-scenes maestros of your sexual journey.

Desire and Hormones: Desire is often influenced by fluctuations in sex hormones like estrogen and testosterone. These hormones can amplify or diminish your interest in sexual activities.

Arousal and Hormones: Hormones play a significant role in preparing your body for arousal. Elevated levels of testosterone can enhance sensitivity and arousal, contributing to the body's readiness for pleasure.

Orgasm and Hormones: The climax of the Female Sexual Response Cycle is marked by a surge of oxytocin, often called the "love hormone." This hormone fosters emotional bonding and intimacy, making orgasms not just physical experiences but emotional ones as well.

Understanding the Menstrual Cycle's Impact

The ebb and flow of desire and arousal is intimately linked to the menstrual cycle, a dance choreographed by hormones that shifts in intensity over the course of the month.

Follicular Phase: As estrogen levels rise after menstruation, many individuals experience an increase in sexual desire and a heightened sensitivity to sexual cues.

Ovulatory Phase: Around ovulation, testosterone levels also peak, contributing to a surge in sexual interest, confidence, and adventurousness.

Luteal Phase: In the latter half of the cycle, progesterone levels increase. Some people might experience a decrease in sexual desire due to hormonal changes and potential mood shifts.

Understanding these patterns can help you embrace the fluctuations in your desire and arousal with greater awareness and acceptance.

Hormone Therapy and Its Effects on Sexual Drive

For some individuals, hormonal imbalances or medical conditions can impact sexual desire. Hormone therapy is a potential avenue for addressing these concerns.

Testosterone Replacement: Testosterone therapy, when prescribed by a medical professional, can help boost sexual desire and arousal in individuals with low testosterone levels.

Hormonal Birth Control: Some forms of birth control can influence sexual desire due to their impact on hormone levels. It's important to communicate openly with your healthcare provider if you experience changes in libido.

Menopause and Hormone Replacement: Menopause brings about significant hormonal changes that can affect sexual response. Hormone replacement therapy can alleviate symptoms and restore some aspects of sexual desire and comfort.

Embracing Hormonal Harmony

As you journey through the realms of desire, arousal, and satisfaction, remember that your body's hormonal symphony is as unique as you are. By understanding the role of hormones, you can gain insights into the rhythms and patterns of your own sexual responses. Whether you're navigating the ups and downs of the menstrual cycle or considering hormone therapy, the key is to embrace your body's natural ebbs and flows.

In the chapters that follow, we'll delve deeper into strategies for harmonizing hormones through lifestyle choices, communication with healthcare providers, and embracing the beauty of your body's unique hormonal dance. With knowledge as your guide, you'll be equipped to navigate the labyrinth of hormones and enhance your sexual well-being, fostering a deep connection between mind, body, and the intricate world of hormones.

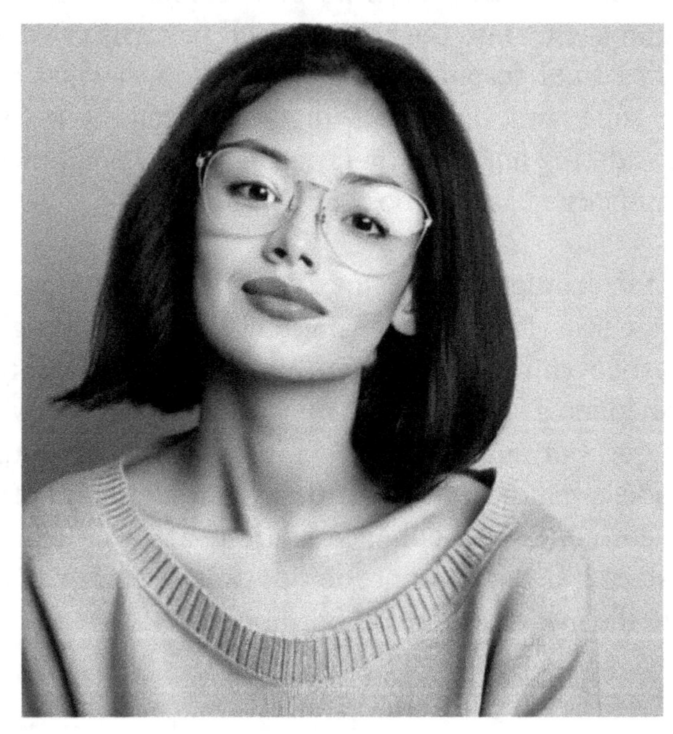

Chapter 4

Enhancing Desire

Communication with Your Partner About Desires

Desire is the spark that ignites the journey through the Female Sexual Response Cycle, and in this chapter, we'll explore how to not only kindle that spark but also fan it into a passionate flame. We'll discuss the vital role of communication with your partner(s) about desires, the liberating world of exploring fantasies and role-play, and how to rediscover passion in long-term relationships. By enhancing desire, you pave the way for a more fulfilling and satisfying sexual experience.

Communication is the cornerstone of any healthy and satisfying sexual relationship. Open, honest, and respectful conversations about your desires are essential for fostering intimacy and understanding.

Creating a Safe Space: Establish a safe and non-judgmental environment where both you and your partner(s) feel comfortable discussing your desires. Trust is the foundation upon which these conversations thrive.

Active Listening: Encourage active listening. Allow your partner(s) to express their desires, needs, and boundaries. This reciprocity fosters a deeper emotional connection.

Asking and Expressing: Don't be afraid to ask for what you want and express your desires. Remember, your partner(s) can't read your mind. Sharing your fantasies and desires can lead to exciting new experiences and deepen intimacy.

Exploring Fantasies and Role-Play

Fantasies are the fertile ground from which desire often springs. They allow you to explore the limitless realms of imagination and desire. Role-play is a liberating way to bring these fantasies to life.

Understanding Fantasies: Fantasies are a natural and healthy part of human sexuality. They can range from the simple and romantic to the bold and adventurous. Recognize and embrace your own fantasies without judgment.

Role-Play: Role-play involves adopting different personas or scenarios to create exciting and novel sexual experiences. It can help you step out of your comfort zone and explore new facets of desire.

Consent and Boundaries: In all aspects of exploring desires and fantasies, consent and boundaries are paramount. Ensure that both you and your partner(s) are comfortable and in agreement with any activities you explore.

Rediscovering Passion in Long-Term Relationships

Long-term relationships can sometimes experience a dwindling of desire. However, with intention and effort, passion can be reignited.

Embrace Novelty: Inject novelty into your relationship by trying new activities together, traveling, or exploring shared interests. New experiences can rekindle desire.

Maintain Emotional Connection: Emotional intimacy is closely linked to desire. Nurture your emotional bond through open communication, quality time together, and acts of love and affection.

Sensate Focus: Engage in sensate focus exercises, which involve non-sexual touching and exploration of each other's bodies. These exercises can help rebuild physical and emotional intimacy.

Enhancing Desire Together
Desire is not a static state but a dynamic force that can be nurtured and enriched. The journey toward enhancing desire is a shared one, best undertaken with a partner(s) who supports and cherishes your desires.

Chapter 5

Igniting Arousal

Physical and Mental Stimulation Techniques

Arousal is the bridge between desire and ecstasy, and it's where your body's responses truly come alive. In this chapter, we'll explore the art of igniting arousal through physical and mental stimulation techniques, the sensual activities that can heighten the experience, and how to address common challenges that may arise on your journey to arousal. By mastering the art of arousal, you'll discover the keys to unlocking intense pleasure and connection.

Arousal involves both physical and mental components, and the synergy between them is where the magic happens.

Physical Stimulation:
Foreplay: Engage in extended foreplay to build anticipation and arousal. Kiss, caress, and explore each other's bodies with intention and desire.

Touch: Experiment with different types of touch, from gentle strokes to firmer pressure. Pay attention to erogenous zones like the neck, breasts, and inner thighs.

Sensory Play: Incorporate sensory play, such as using silk scarves or feathers, to awaken your senses and heighten sensitivity.

Mental Stimulation:

Fantasy: Allow your imagination to run wild with sexual fantasies. Create scenarios and narratives that arouse your desires and share them with your partner(s).

Erotic Literature and Media: Reading erotic literature or watching sensual films can stimulate your mind and ignite arousal. Discussing these experiences with your partner(s) can also be a form of foreplay.

Mindfulness and Presence: Practice mindfulness during sexual encounters. Being fully present in the moment, focusing on sensations and emotions, can intensify arousal.

Exploring Sensual Activities to Heighten Arousal

Sensual activities offer a diverse array of pathways to heightened arousal and pleasure.

Massage: Sensual massages can be both relaxing and intensely arousing. Use scented oils and take turns massaging each other's bodies, paying close attention to erogenous zones.

Sensual Dance: Experiment with sensual dance, either alone or with your partner(s). The act of moving your body in a seductive manner can ignite arousal and boost confidence.

Food Play: Incorporate food into your sexual activities. Experiment with temperature play using ice cubes or indulge in a shared dessert, using your bodies as the utensils.

Exploration of Kinks and Fetishes: If you and your partner(s) are open to it, explore kinks and fetishes that align with your desires. Consent and communication are paramount in this realm.

Addressing Common Challenges in Achieving Arousal

Arousal can sometimes be elusive, but understanding common challenges can help you navigate them.

Stress: Stress can inhibit arousal. Practice stress-reduction techniques such as deep breathing, meditation, or yoga.

Distraction: Our busy lives can be distracting. Create a space for intimacy that is free from distractions like phones or work-related thoughts.

Performance Anxiety: Anxiety about sexual performance can hinder arousal. Communicate with your partner(s) about any anxieties and remember that sex is about connection, not just performance.

Physical Factors: Physical factors, such as medication or medical conditions, can affect arousal. Consult with a healthcare professional if you suspect any underlying issues.

The Call to Action: Ignite Arousal

Arousal is a dynamic state that can be cultivated through intention, exploration, and communication. As you journey through this chapter, remember that the path to heightened arousal is a personal one, unique to you and your partner(s). It's about discovering what ignites your desires and stoking the flames of passion.

Now, take action by exploring physical and mental stimulation techniques, indulging in sensual activities, and addressing any challenges that may arise. The pursuit of heightened arousal is a journey of self-discovery and connection, a journey that promises to bring you closer to the electric sensations and intense pleasure that await you on the path to ecstasy.

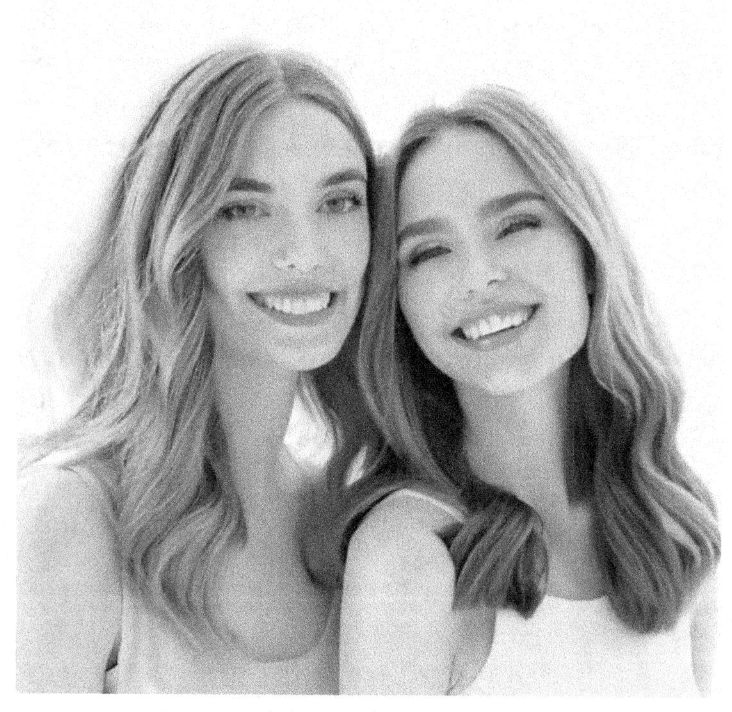

Chapter 6

Climaxing with Orgasm

Understanding the Anatomy of Female Orgasm

Orgasm is the climactic crescendo of the Female Sexual Response Cycle, an explosion of pleasure that embodies the essence of sexual fulfillment. In this chapter, we will delve into the intricate anatomy of the female orgasm, explore techniques to achieve this pinnacle of pleasure, and provide guidance on overcoming orgasmic difficulties. By understanding the nuances of the orgasmic experience, you'll be equipped to embrace the full spectrum of ecstasy.

The female orgasm is a symphony of physiological and psychological sensations, an intricate interplay between the body and the mind.

Physiological Changes: During orgasm, the body undergoes rhythmic contractions of the pelvic floor muscles. These contractions release built-up sexual tension and result in intense pleasurable sensations.

The Clitoris and G-Spot: The clitoris is a highly sensitive organ rich in nerve endings. Stimulation of the clitoris is a common pathway to orgasm. The G-spot, an erogenous zone located within the vaginal wall, can also contribute to intense orgasms for some individuals.

Vaginal and Uterine Contractions: The walls of the vagina and uterus contract rhythmically during orgasm, contributing to the waves of pleasure. These contractions are involuntary and a key hallmark of orgasm.

Techniques for Achieving Orgasm

The journey to orgasm is as varied as the individuals embarking upon it. Exploring different techniques can enhance your understanding of what brings you to climax.

Clitoral Stimulation: Many individuals find clitoral stimulation to be the most reliable pathway to orgasm. Experiment with different types of touch, pressure, and speeds to discover what works best for you.

Vaginal Stimulation: G-spot stimulation through penetration can lead to intense orgasms for some. Experiment with angles, positions, and rhythms to find what feels most pleasurable.

Combination Stimulation: Combining clitoral and vaginal stimulation can create a powerful synergy of pleasure. This can be achieved through manual stimulation, oral sex, or the use of sex toys.

Overcoming Orgasmic Difficulties

Orgasmic difficulties are common and can stem from various factors. Addressing these challenges can pave the way to a more fulfilling sexual experience.

Relaxation and Mindset: Creating a relaxed and comfortable environment is essential for reaching orgasm. Let go of performance pressure and focus on the sensations and emotional connection.

Communication: Openly communicate with your partner(s) about your desires, needs, and any difficulties you may be facing. Partners can provide support and understanding during this journey.

Exploration and Self-Discovery: Explore your own body through self-pleasure. Self-discovery can enhance your knowledge of what brings you pleasure and makes it easier to communicate your needs to your partner(s).

Professional Help: If difficulties persist, consider seeking guidance from a sex therapist or healthcare professional. They can help uncover underlying factors and provide tailored solutions.

Embracing Orgasmic Bliss
The orgasmic experience is as unique as you are, and understanding the elements that contribute to it is a journey of empowerment and self-discovery. As you navigate through this chapter, remember that the pursuit of orgasm is not about a specific destination; it's about embracing the journey of exploration, communication, and self-awareness.

Now, take the insights from this chapter and put them into action. Explore different techniques, communicate openly with your partner(s), and remember that the path to orgasm is one of pleasure, connection, and embracing the waves of ecstasy that come with embracing your own body's responses.

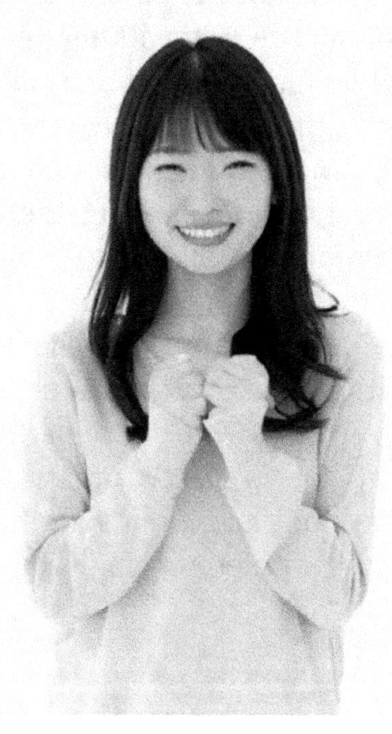

Chapter 7

Embracing the Afterglow

The Importance of Post-Orgasmic Bonding

The afterglow of sexual intimacy is a serene and profound space where the echoes of pleasure continue to resonate. In this chapter, we'll explore the importance of post-orgasmic bonding, the role of self-care and relaxation after sexual activity, and the ways in which you can strengthen emotional intimacy with your partner(s). By embracing the afterglow, you can deepen your connection with both yourself and your partner(s), nurturing the emotional aspects of your sexual journey.

Orgasm is not merely a physical release; it's a gateway to emotional intimacy and connection. The moments after climax offer a unique opportunity for bonding and reflection.

Oxytocin Release: During orgasm, the body releases oxytocin, often called the "love hormone." This hormone fosters emotional bonding and trust, deepening the connection between you and your partner(s).

Emotional Vulnerability: Post-orgasm, individuals often experience a sense of emotional vulnerability and openness. This can be a valuable time for communication and deeper connection.

Mutual Satisfaction: Sharing the afterglow can be a testament to the satisfaction and pleasure experienced during sexual activity, reinforcing the connection and mutual fulfillment.

Self-Care and Relaxation After Sexual Activity

After the intensity of sexual activity, self-care and relaxation are essential for both physical and emotional well-being.

Rest and Recovery: Give your body time to recover. Physical rest is important, especially if your sexual encounter was physically demanding.

Hydration: Staying hydrated is crucial, as sexual activity can lead to dehydration. Drinking water can also help flush out toxins and promote a sense of well-being.

Comfort: Create a comfortable space for post-sex relaxation. Soft lighting, cozy blankets, and calming music can enhance the experience.

Mental Decompression: Take time for mental decompression. Engage in activities that help you unwind and shift your focus from sexual intensity to relaxation.

Strengthening Emotional Intimacy with Your Partner

The afterglow is an ideal time to strengthen emotional intimacy with your partner(s), fostering a deeper connection.

Cuddle and Communicate: Cuddling and sharing your thoughts and feelings in the post-orgasmic state can be incredibly intimate. Use this time to express your affection and appreciation for each other.

Express Gratitude: Take a moment to express gratitude for the shared experience. This simple act of appreciation can deepen emotional bonds.

Reflect and Connect: Reflect on the sexual encounter and discuss what you both enjoyed. This communication not only enhances intimacy but also guides future encounters.

Plan for Future Intimacy: Use the afterglow as an opportunity to plan for future sexual encounters or intimate activities, building anticipation and excitement.

Embrace the Afterglow

The afterglow is a magical realm where the physical and emotional aspects of your sexual journey harmonize. It's a time for connection, reflection, and nurturing the bonds with your partner(s).

As you explore the significance of post-orgasmic bonding, self-care, and emotional intimacy, remember that these moments are precious and should be cherished. Take action by actively engaging in the afterglow, whether through cuddling, conversation, or shared moments of relaxation. The afterglow is a testament to the power of intimacy and connection, reminding you that the journey of sexual fulfillment extends far beyond the climax, into the serene and beautiful space where you and your partner(s) can embrace the depth of your emotions and desires.

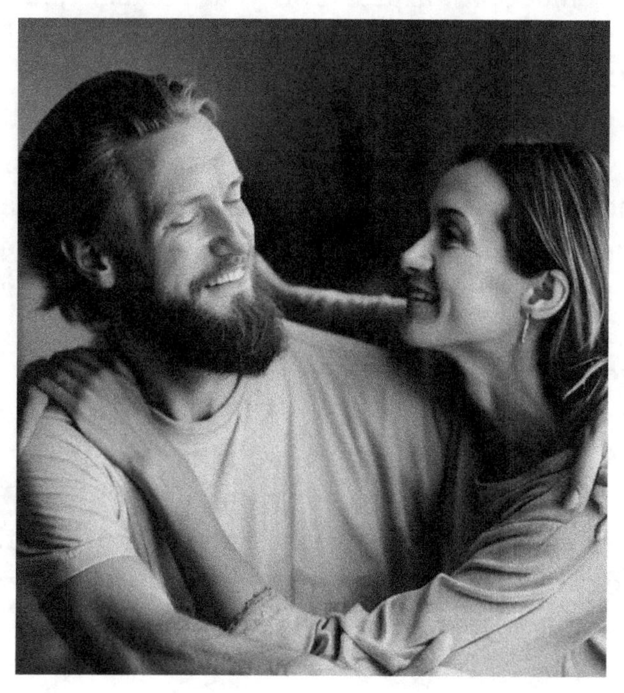

Chapter 8

Factors Affecting Sexual Response

Age and Sexual Response

The symphony of the Female Sexual Response Cycle is influenced by a multitude of factors, both internal and external. In this chapter, we'll delve into three significant factors, age, medical conditions, and trauma, and their impact on sexual response. By understanding how these factors interact with your body's natural rhythms, you'll be better equipped to navigate challenges and cultivate a fulfilling sexual well-being.

The passage of time brings about changes in the body and the way it responds to sexual stimuli.

Desire and Age: Desire can evolve over time. Factors such as hormonal changes and life circumstances can influence sexual desire. Embrace the shifts and communicate openly with your partner(s) about changing needs.

Arousal and Age: The physical response to arousal, such as lubrication and blood flow, might change with age. Communication and exploration become essential to adapt to these changes.

Orgasm and Age: While some individuals might experience changes in orgasmic intensity with age, others might find that experience deepens as they grow more attuned to their bodies.

Medical Conditions and Medications

Medical conditions and medications can have profound effects on sexual response.

Chronic Illness: Conditions such as diabetes, heart disease, and chronic pain can affect sexual desire, arousal, and physical capability. Consulting with healthcare professionals can help manage these challenges.

Medications: Certain medications, including antidepressants, blood pressure medications, and hormonal treatments, can impact sexual desire, arousal, and orgasmic response. Discuss potential side effects with your healthcare provider.

Communication: Openly communicate with your healthcare provider about any sexual concerns related to medical conditions or medications. They can offer guidance and explore potential solutions.

Trauma and Its Impact on Sexual Well-Being

Past trauma, whether physical or emotional, can significantly influence sexual well-being.

Psychological Impact: Trauma can create emotional barriers to sexual desire and intimacy. Feelings of anxiety, fear, or guilt can hinder the ability to fully engage in sexual activities.

Physical Impact: Physical trauma, such as surgery or injury, can affect the body's response to sexual stimuli. Sensations might change, requiring exploration and communication to adapt to new sensations.

Seeking Support: If trauma is affecting your sexual well-being, consider seeking support from a therapist, counselor, or support group. Addressing emotional and psychological healing is a vital step.

Navigating Influences on Sexual Response

Your sexual response is a dynamic interplay of internal and external factors. By acknowledging the influence of age, medical conditions and medications, and past trauma, you pave the way for a journey of adaptation, exploration, and self-compassion.

Chapter 9

Cultivating a Positive Sexual Identity

Embracing Your Unique Sexual Self

Your sexual identity is a vibrant tapestry woven from your desires, preferences, and beliefs. In this chapter, we'll explore how to cultivate a positive sexual identity by embracing your unique self, challenging societal norms and expectations, and fostering a healthy and empowered relationship with your sexuality. By embarking on this journey of self-discovery and acceptance, you can create a harmonious connection between your inner desires and your external expression.

Each person's sexual identity is as unique as a fingerprint, and it's a mosaic composed of myriad elements.

Self-Exploration: Take time to explore your desires, boundaries, and preferences. Self-pleasure can be a powerful tool for understanding your body and what brings you pleasure.

Communication: Openly communicate with your partner(s) about your sexual desires, needs, and boundaries. Shared understanding and mutual respect are the foundation of a positive sexual identity.

Self-Acceptance: Embrace yourself without judgment. Your sexual identity is a beautiful part of who you are. Acceptance and self-love are the cornerstones of a positive journey.

Challenging Societal Norms and Expectations

Society often imposes norms and expectations on sexual identity. Challenging these constructs is essential for cultivating a positive sense of self.

Questioning Assumptions: Challenge assumptions about what is "normal" or "acceptable." Remember that there is no one-size-fits-all definition of a positive sexual identity.

Breaking Taboos: Engage in conversations that challenge taboos and stigma around sexuality. By dismantling these barriers, you contribute to a more inclusive and understanding society.

Media Literacy: Be mindful of media influences that may shape your perceptions of sexual identity. Question unrealistic portrayals and seek diverse representations.

Fostering a Healthy and Empowered Sexual Identity

A healthy and empowered sexual identity is one that aligns with your values and promotes well-being.

Consent and Boundaries: Prioritize consent and boundaries in all sexual interactions. Respecting your own boundaries and those of others is integral to a positive identity.

Education: Educate yourself about sexual health, pleasure, and consent. Knowledge is empowering and can help you make informed decisions about your body and relationships.

Seek Support: If you're navigating challenges related to your sexual identity, consider seeking support from friends, partners, therapists, or support groups. You're not alone on this journey.

Cultivating Your Unique Identity
Your sexual identity is a canvas waiting for your unique brushstrokes. As you embark on this chapter, remember that embracing your desires, challenging norms, and fostering empowerment are integral to cultivating a positive sexual identity.

Chapter 10

The Role of Communication

Open Dialogue with Your Partner About Sexual Needs

Communication is the cornerstone of a vibrant and fulfilling sexual relationship. In this chapter, we'll explore the pivotal role of open dialogue with your partner about sexual needs, and when necessary, seeking professional help to navigate challenges that arise. By honing the art of communication, you'll forge deeper connections, enhance intimacy, and overcome obstacles together.

Effective communication is the bedrock upon which satisfying sexual relationships are built.

Creating a Safe Space: Establish an environment where open communication is not only welcomed but encouraged. Both you and your partner(s) should feel safe expressing desires, boundaries, and concerns.

Regular Check-Ins: Regularly check in with each other about your sexual experiences and desires. Open the lines of communication to ensure that both you and your partner(s) feel heard and understood.

Active Listening: Be an active listener when your partner(s) communicates their needs. Show empathy and validate their feelings.

Expressing Desires and Boundaries: Share your desires and boundaries with your partner(s). This mutual understanding can enhance intimacy and lead to more fulfilling sexual experiences.

Seeking Professional Help When Communication Breaks Down

Communication breakdowns can occur, but seeking professional help can be transformative for your relationship.

Counseling or Therapy: If communication becomes difficult, consider couples counseling or therapy. A trained professional can facilitate conversations and provide tools for effective communication.

Sex Therapy: Sex therapy is specifically focused on addressing sexual concerns and improving sexual well-being. A sex therapist can guide you through discussions about desire, satisfaction, and overcoming challenges.

Unresolved Conflicts: If communication becomes a source of unresolved conflicts, seeking professional help early can prevent the issues from escalating.

Mastering the Art of Communication
Communication is the bridge that connects you and your partner(s), fostering emotional intimacy and deeper connections. As you navigate through this chapter, remember that open dialogue about sexual needs is not just a skill, it's an ongoing commitment to nurturing your relationship.

Take action by engaging in regular conversations about sexual desires, boundaries, and experiences. Approach these discussions with empathy, respect, and a genuine desire to understand and support your partner(s). If you encounter challenges in communication, don't hesitate to seek professional help. Trained therapists can offer guidance, provide tools, and create a safe space for addressing difficult topics.

Remember that the art of communication is a journey, one that requires patience, understanding, and a willingness to learn and grow together. By embracing communication as a foundation for your sexual relationship, you pave the way for a dynamic and enduring bond that can weather challenges and celebrate shared joys.

Chapter 11

Navigating Challenges

Overcoming Relationship Hurdles Impacting Sexual Desire

The path to a fulfilling and satisfying sexual journey is not always smooth; challenges can arise that test your resilience and connection. In this chapter, we'll navigate through common obstacles that many individuals face. We'll explore overcoming relationship hurdles impacting sexual desire, dealing with body image issues and insecurities, and strategies for reviving a diminished sex drive. By meeting these challenges with understanding and proactive approaches, you can foster a resilient and vibrant sexual well-being.

Relationships can experience ups and downs that impact sexual desire. Addressing these hurdles can strengthen your bond.

Communication: Openly discuss any relationship concerns. Explore any emotional barriers that might be affecting your sexual connection.

Quality Time: Spend quality time together outside of sexual activities. Emotional intimacy can lay the foundation for a healthy sexual relationship.

Rediscovering Intimacy: Engage in activities that foster emotional intimacy, such as cuddling, sharing secrets, or simply enjoying each other's company.

Dealing with Body Image Issues and Insecurities

Body image issues and insecurities can hinder sexual confidence. Embracing self-acceptance is essential.

Positive Self-Talk: Replace negative self-talk with positive affirmations. Celebrate your body for its uniqueness and the pleasure it brings.

Sensual Exploration: Engage in sensual activities that celebrate your body's sensations. Sensate focus exercises and self-pleasure can help you reconnect with your body.

Intimacy with the Lights On: Experiment with keeping the lights on during sexual activities. This can foster a greater sense of vulnerability and intimacy.

Strategies for Reviving Diminished Sex Drive

A diminished sex drive can be a temporary challenge. Employing strategies can help reignite desire.

Prioritize Self-Care: Address stressors in your life and engage in self-care practices that promote relaxation and emotional well-being.

Explore Fantasy: Allow your imagination to reignite desire. Explore new fantasies or revisit old ones to kindle the flame of passion.

Date Nights: Plan regular date nights to focus on your connection. Shared experiences and quality time can rejuvenate your bond.

Seek Professional Advice: If a diminished sex drive persists, consider seeking guidance from a healthcare provider or sex therapist to identify potential underlying causes and solutions.

Conquering Challenges Together
Challenges are a natural part of any journey, and your sexual journey is no exception. As you navigate through this chapter, remember that challenges can be opportunities for growth and transformation.

Take action by addressing relationship hurdles with open communication and fostering emotional intimacy. Embrace your body and confront insecurities with self-love and acceptance. If you're facing a diminished sex drive, employ strategies that resonate with you, and seek professional help if needed.

Remember, your journey is unique, and your ability to face challenges together is a testament to your commitment and resilience. By confronting challenges head-on, you foster a sexual well-being that is adaptable, enduring, and filled with shared triumphs.

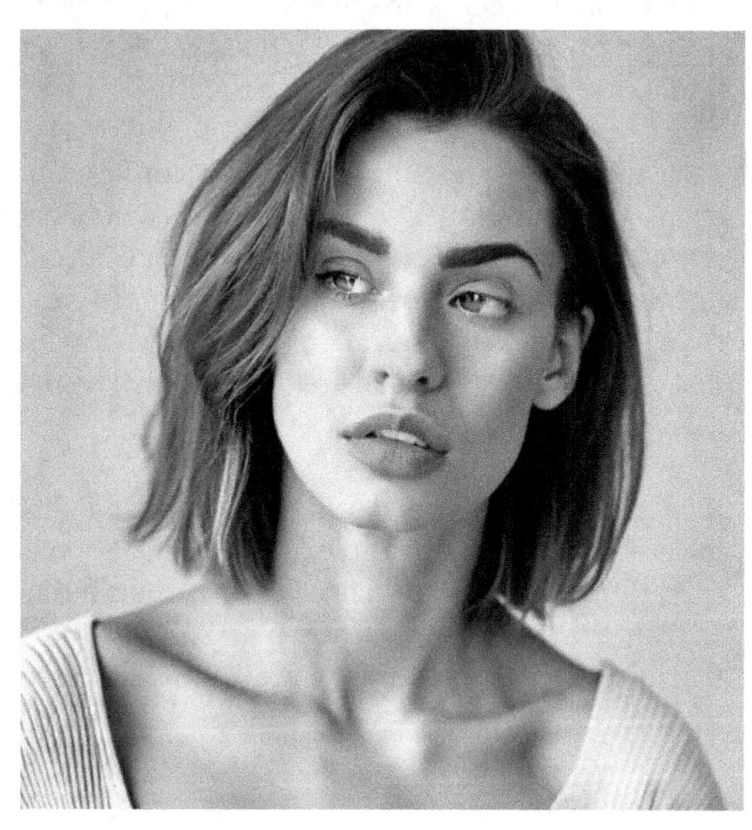

Chapter 12

The Journey to Long-Term Fulfillment

Developing a Lifelong Connection with Your Sexual Response

A fulfilling sexual journey is not a destination; it's a lifelong odyssey of self-discovery, connection, and growth. In this final chapter, we'll explore how to develop a lifelong connection with your sexual response, the importance of continual exploration and adaptation, and how to embrace change and growth in your sexual journey. By embarking on this journey to long-term fulfillment, you'll discover that the greatest rewards lie not in the destination, but in the ever-evolving adventure itself.

Your sexual response is an intricate symphony unique to you. Developing a lifelong connection involves nurturing and understanding it throughout the years.

Self-Awareness: As you evolve, stay attuned to changes in desire, arousal, and satisfaction. Embrace the shifts with self-awareness and adapt to your body's rhythms.

Communication: Continue open dialogue with your partner(s). Share your desires and listen to theirs. As your desires evolve, these conversations ensure that your connection remains strong.

Continual Exploration and Adaptation

Exploration is the fuel that keeps your sexual journey vibrant and exciting. Never stop seeking new pathways to pleasure and connection.

New Experiences: Seek out new experiences that challenge your comfort zone. Experiment with different activities, scenarios, or even locations to keep the journey fresh.

Evolve Together: As individuals and relationships grow, sexual dynamics can change. Embrace this evolution and adapt together, finding new ways to connect.

Embracing Change and Growth in Your Sexual Journey

Change is an inevitable part of life, and it's no different in your sexual journey. Embrace the ebb and flow of change with an open heart.

Life Transitions: Major life transitions, such as parenthood or career changes, can impact your sexual journey. Approach these transitions as opportunities for growth and adaptation.

Aging: With age comes physical and emotional changes. Embrace these changes as natural progressions and find new ways to experience pleasure and intimacy.

Embrace the Eternal Journey

Your sexual journey is a tapestry woven from desires, experiences, and emotions, a journey that is uniquely yours. As you navigate through this chapter, remember that long-term fulfillment is not about reaching a finish line; it's about embracing the eternal journey of growth and connection.

Take action by fostering a lifelong connection with your sexual response. Continually explore new horizons of pleasure, both individually and with your partner(s). Embrace change with grace and an understanding that your sexual journey, like life itself, is a fluid and evolving experience.

In each moment, whether during the peaks of passion or the quiet afterglow, remember that your journey to long-term fulfillment is a tribute to your resilience, curiosity, and capacity for love and connection. By embracing this journey, you infuse your life with a richness that knows no bounds, a fulfillment that extends far beyond the pages of this book and into the tapestry of your own uniquely beautiful sexual journey.

Conclusion

In the pages of this book, we've embarked on a journey through the intricate landscape of the Female Sexual Response Cycle, a journey that has illuminated the pathways to understanding, empowerment, and fulfillment. From the flames of desire to the pinnacle of ecstasy, your body is a canvas painted with the colors of pleasure and connection.

As you close this chapter of exploration, it's essential to reflect on the profound potential that lies within your Sexual Response Cycle. Your desires, your body, and your journey are uniquely yours, and they deserve to be honored, celebrated, and embraced.

Empowered Steps to Enhancing Your Sex Drive

To enhance your sex drive is to honor the vitality of your own desires and the beauty of your body's responses. It's a journey that takes courage, understanding, and a commitment to self-discovery.

Here are some empowered steps to guide you:

1. Embrace Self-Discovery: Your journey begins with self-discovery. Take time to understand your desires, preferences, and boundaries. Explore your body through self-pleasure and open communication with your partner(s).

2. Prioritize Communication: Open and honest communication is the cornerstone of a vibrant sexual relationship. Regularly engage in conversations about desires, boundaries, and experiences.

3. Cultivate Emotional Intimacy: Emotional intimacy is the key to unlocking the full potential of your Sexual Response Cycle. Nurture emotional bonds with your partner(s) through quality time, trust, and shared experiences.

4. Challenge Societal Norms: Challenge societal norms and expectations that may limit your sexual identity. Embrace your uniqueness, reject unrealistic beauty standards, and celebrate diversity in all its forms.

5. Navigate Challenges Together: Challenges are part of every journey. Face them with resilience and proactive approaches. Address relationship hurdles, body image issues, and diminished sex drive with empathy and communication.

6. Seek Professional Help When Needed: If you encounter persistent challenges, do not hesitate to seek professional guidance. Sex therapists, counselors, and healthcare providers can offer valuable insights and solutions.

7. Embrace Self-Love: Above all, practice self-love and self-acceptance. Celebrate your body, your desires, and your journey. Your sexual well-being is a reflection of your self-worth and self-compassion.

In closing, your journey through the Female Sexual Response Cycle is a testament to the power of self-discovery, connection, and the boundless potential for pleasure and fulfillment. By embracing the uniqueness of your desires and the beauty of your body's responses, you embark on a journey of self-empowerment and sexual well-being that knows no limits.

May your path be filled with pleasure, passion, and the deep connection that arises from understanding and embracing the depths of your own sexual response.